Nature's Wisdom

Awakening Consciousness Through Natural Connection

Kim Aronson

Acknowledgements

Thank you to S. F. Wilson for the amazing editing of this book. If you need a reliable editor, you can contact her at sfbk.editing@gmail.com

Thank you, Rosy, for always being willing to point me in the right direction.

Dedication

To the nature lover we all carry inside.

A rose in bloom, a symphony of color and fragrance composed in the heart of a wild garden, reveals nature's artistry.

Epigraph

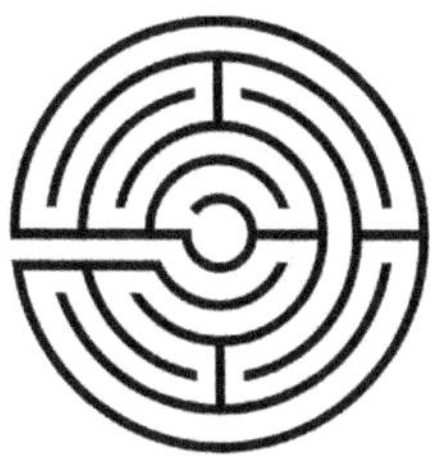

The privilege of a lifetime is to become who you truly are
- C. G. Jung

Contents

All Wisdom Manuals

All The Books in The Wisdom Manuals series:

The Conscious Caregiver's Compass
- Caring for Your Aging Parent

Reflections of the Heart
- A Journey Through Love Addiction

The Tapestry of Grief
- A Journey Through Loss

Navigating Divorce
- A Path Toward Transformation

Bridging the Relationship Void
- From Loneliness to Connection

The Sensitive Soul
- The Hidden Power of Your Empathy

Nature's Wisdom

Sign up for the newsletter to be notified of new books and receive exclusive offers!

www.wisdommanuals.com/newsletter

Books That Bring Awareness, Compassion & Insights Into Your Everyday Life
www.WisdomManuals.com

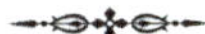

My professional website is: www.KimAronson.com
I offer intuitive readings to illuminate your path and provide clarity, personalized coaching sessions designed to empower you to reach your goals, and insightful teachings that will deepen your understanding of yourself and the world around you.

Wisdom Groups

Join today

Wisdom Groups For Contemplation & Conversation
A space for support, genuine reflection and deep discussion

Many of us feel a deep sense of disconnection in the face of life's challenges—from ourselves, others, and a meaningful purpose. Whether it's the grief of loss, the stress of everyday life, the pain of heartbreak, or the uncertainty of the future, these experiences often leave us feeling isolated, lost and longing for deeper understanding and connection.

Wisdom Groups are online Zoom groups inspired by this Wisdom Manuals book series. They are dedicated to bringing awareness, compassion and insights into everyday life, and offer a supportive environment to explore our shared struggles, reflect together, and transform pain into growth.

What to Expect in a Wisdom Group:

- **Weekly Gatherings:** Each session of 75 minutes begins with a topic or passage from one of the Wisdom Manuals books for contemplation, followed by group sharing and discussion.

- **Facilitated Conversations:** I'll guide our discussions to create a safe space for open sharing, reflection and mutual support. We'll explore awareness, consciousness and empathy as sources of strength to integrate wisdom into our everyday lives.

- **Planting Seeds Together:** Through shared reflections, we'll grow as a community by turning emotional pain into opportunities for self-discovery and deeper connection.

The inspiration for the Wisdom Manuals book series comes from my lifelong journey of questioning: Why are we here? How do we find meaning in our struggles? What can we learn from the difficult moments in life? Through creativity, personal experiences and spiritual exploration, I've discovered just how much wisdom can be embodied in our daily lives when we connect with others and face our challenges with an open heart.

Is This Group for You?

If you're feeling:

- Disconnected from yourself or others, yearning for a deeper connection
- Overwhelmed by everyday life
- Stuck in stress, anxiety or grief, needing a way forward
- Lonely or uncertain about your path in life, seeking a sense of meaning and belonging
- Curious about how to turn life's challenges into empowering growth

opportunities

Then a Wisdom Group can offer you a community and tools for deeper self-awareness, connection and transformation.

Join us as we explore, reflect, and grow—one meaningful conversation at a time.

For more information or to join a Wisdom Group, visit: https://ww w.wisdommanuals.com/wisdom-groups

Introduction

In the hustle of modern life, we often lose touch with our true selves and the world around us. Yet, nestled within the embrace of nature lies a profound pathway to self-discovery, growth, and heightened consciousness. This book invites you on an extraordinary journey—one that will lead you back to your authentic self through the timeless wisdom of the natural world.

Imagine standing atop a mountain, feeling the crisp air fill your lungs as you gaze upon vast horizons. Picture yourself beside a babbling brook, its gentle song soothing your spirit and washing away the noise of daily life. Envision walking through an ancient forest, where towering trees whisper secrets of resilience and interconnection. These are not mere experiences—they are gateways to a deeper understanding of who you truly are.

Within these pages, you'll discover how nature serves as a mirror, reflecting the hidden depths of your psyche and illuminating paths to personal transformation. You'll learn to read the subtle language of the earth, finding profound meaning in the dance of leaves, the flight of birds, and the cycles of the seasons. Through myths, exercises, and reflections, you'll explore powerful concepts like archetypes, synchronicity, and the interplay of masculine and feminine energies—all through the lens of our relationship with the natural world.

This book is more than a guide; it's an invitation to awaken; to shed the layers of societal expectations and reconnect with your core essence; and to find balance, purpose, and a renewed sense of wonder. Whether you're a seasoned nature enthusiast or someone yearning to escape the concrete jungle, these pages hold transformative potential for all who seek a more conscious way of being.

Prepare to embark on a journey that will change how you see yourself, others, and the world around you. Welcome to the adventure of awakening to nature's wisdom.

Chapter One

Ego Exploration

The ego, our sense of self and identity, plays a crucial role in how we perceive and interact with the world around us. When we immerse ourselves in nature, we open up opportunities for profound self-reflection and growth. By engaging with the natural world, we can gain insights into our own behaviors, thoughts, and emotions. This process of becoming more self-aware through our experiences in nature can lead to personal growth and more harmonious relationships.

The Stony Path

In a tranquil valley filled with colorful wildflowers, there was a towering mountain known as the Ego Peak. Many villagers believed that climbing to its summit would grant them life-long wisdom. A young man named Kiran was determined to conquer the peak, thinking that success would solidify his identity.

As Kiran ascended the rocky path, he faced harsh winds and slippery stones. He felt frustrated as he struggled against the mountain's challenges. In a moment of exhaustion, he sat on a boulder and closed his eyes, surrendering his quest for identity. Instead of striving to prove himself, he began to listen to the rustling leaves and the chirping birds. In that silence, he discovered that the wisdom he sought was not in conquering the mountain but in appreciating the journey itself.

When Kiran finally reached the summit, he saw not just his reflection in the clouds but a vast landscape connecting him to all beings. He realized that the ego was a part of him but did not define him—the journey did.

Reflection

This story illustrates that the ego, while a part of our identity, does not comprise our whole self. Engaging with nature can prompt moments of surrender and reflection, allowing us to redefine our understanding of self-worth beyond perceived achievements.

Exercises

1. Nature's Mirror

This exercise encourages us to observe similarities between natural formations and aspects of our ego. By drawing parallels between ourselves and nature, we can gain insights into our personality, strengths, and areas for growth. This practice helps foster a deeper connection with the natural world while promoting self-reflection and awareness.

Find a comfortable spot in nature and spend at least 30 minutes observing your surroundings. Look for elements in the landscape that resonate with aspects of your ego or personality. For example, you might feel strong and grounded like a mountain, or fluid and changing like a river. Take note of these connections and write about them in a journal. Reflect on how these natural elements embody qualities you admire or aspire to develop within yourself.

Example: During a hike, Sarah noticed a resilient pine tree growing from a rocky cliff face. She realized this mirrored her own determination in the face of challenges. The tree's ability to thrive in harsh conditions inspired her to embrace difficulties as opportunities for growth. This observation helped Sarah recognize and appreciate her own resilience, boosting her self-awareness and confidence.

2. Gratitude Nature Ritual

This exercise aims to cultivate gratitude towards nature, which can help shift our perspective and reduce the ego's sense of self-importance. By expressing thankfulness for the natural world, we can foster a deeper connection to something greater than ourselves, promoting humility and a more balanced sense of self.

Find a quiet outdoor setting and sit comfortably. Spend 10 minutes expressing gratitude to the natural elements around you. Thank the trees for providing oxygen, the soil for supporting life, the sun for its warmth and energy, and any other aspects of nature you observe. If possible, speak your gratitude aloud. Notice how this practice impacts your sense of self and your connection to the world around you. After the exercise, journal about your experience and any insights you gained.

Example: Mark practiced this ritual in his backyard, thanking the grass for its softness, the birds for their songs, and the breeze for its refreshing touch. As he expressed gratitude, he felt his usual stress and self-centeredness melt away. Mark realized how interconnected he was with nature, fostering a sense of belonging and humility that stayed with him throughout the day.

3. Seasonal Ego Reflection Ceremony

This exercise encourages regular self-reflection in harmony with nature's cycles. By aligning our introspection with the changing seasons, we can gain insights into our personal growth and the evolving nature of our ego. This practice helps us become more aware of our changing selves and foster a deeper connection with the natural world.

At each seasonal change (the beginnings of spring, summer, autumn, and winter), perform a reflection ritual. Choose a natural setting and spend time meditating on how your ego has shifted during the past season. Gather natural items that represent this seasonal change, such as leaves, stones, or flowers.

Next, create a small altar with these collected items and write your reflections in a journal. Consider how your sense of self, your goals, and your relationships have evolved throughout the past few months. Store your writings and a few of the gathered items for future reference, creating a personal archive of your growth.

Example: During her autumn reflection, Constance collected colorful fallen leaves to represent the changes in her life. She realized that, over the last season or so, her ego had become less rigid, much like the trees shedding their leaves. Emma wrote about how she'd learned to let go of outdated self-perceptions, allowing for new growth. This ceremony helped her recognize and celebrate her personal evolution, inspiring continued self-awareness.

Altering Our Attitude

American philosopher and psychologist William James said, "The greatest discovery of my generation is that a human being can alter his life by altering his attitude." This quote emphasizes the power of perception and mindset in shaping one's identity and experiences. It aligns with the exploration of the ego by highlighting how self-assertion and confidence can transform one's life and relationships.

Chapter Two

The Masks That Make Us

Persona Awareness

T he concept of "the persona" offers a powerful lens through which we can explore our relationship with nature and ourselves. By examining the various roles we play in the different aspects of our lives, we can become more conscious of how these personas influence our interactions with the natural world. As we engage with nature, we have the opportunity to shed the layers of our social masks and connect with our authentic selves, fostering greater self-awareness and personal growth.

The Costumes of the Forest

In a lush forest in a land far away, each forest creature wore a unique costume that reflected the role it wished to play in its community. One gentle rabbit, named Liara, donned a fierce fox costume, believing she needed to appear strong to fit in with the others. At first, this persona intimidated many, but inside, she felt lonely and misunderstood.

One day, while exploring the depths of the woods, Liara stumbled upon a clearing where a wise old owl was perched on a branch. The owl gazed not at her costume but directly at her heart.

"Why wear a mask that is not yours? he asked, confused.

She answered, "To be accepted."

The owl invited Liara to remove her costume and connect with her true self. Hesitantly, Liara shed the heavy fox skin, and as she did, she felt a wave of lightness and freedom wash over her. In her authentic form, she danced among the flowers, re-discovering the joy in being herself. Soon, other animals joined her, shedding their own costumes and celebrating their true selves.

Reflection

This myth highlights the discontinuity that often exists between our personas and authentic selves. Nature provides a safe space for individuals to explore their true identity, reminding us that genuine connections spark when we embrace who we truly are.

Exercises

1. Persona Inventory Journal

This exercise encourages self-reflection by identifying the different roles we play in various aspects of our life. By examining how these personas shift in natural settings, we can gain insight into our authentic self and how nature influences our behavior.

Create a list of the different personas you embody in various aspects of your life (e.g., professional, social, familial). Reflect on how each persona feels when you are in these urban/social/daily scenarios. Write about each persona, describing its characteristics, behaviors, and how it feels to embody that role.

Then, imagine how each persona might react in a *natural* setting. Notice any differences in behavior, thoughts, or emotions. Consider which personas feel more authentic or comfortable in nature and which feel inauthentic or out of place.

Example: Adam, a marketing executive, realized his "professional persona" felt rigid and guarded in the office but relaxed and curious when he took work calls in the park. His "social butterfly persona" thrived at parties but felt unnecessary during solo hikes. By contrasting these experiences, Adam gained insight into which aspects of himself felt most authentic in natural settings.

2. Persona Walk in Nature

This exercise allows you to actively explore how different personas influence our experience of nature. By consciously embodying a specific role during our nature walk, we can observe how it affects our perceptions, emotions, and interactions with the environment.

Choose a persona that you'd like to explore further or one that feels different from your usual self in nature. Go for a walk in a natural setting while consciously embodying this specific persona (e.g., a confident adventurer or a serene healer). Reflect on how this persona influences your interactions with the environment around you and any shifts in perspective you experience.

As you walk, fully embody this persona, adopting its posture, mindset, and way of moving through the world. Pay attention to how this role affects your observations, feelings, and interactions with your surroundings. Notice any new insights or experiences that arise from this perspective.

After your walk, journal about your experience, reflecting on how this persona enhanced or limited your connection with nature and yourself.

Example: Millie, usually cautious in nature, decided to embody a "fearless explorer" persona during a forest hike. She found herself venturing off the main trail, discovering hidden viewpoints, and feeling a surge of confidence. This experience helped Millie realize how her usual persona limited her experiences in nature and inspired her to cultivate more courage in her outdoor adventures.

3. Persona Integration and Affirmation

This exercise helps us integrate various aspects of our personality through positive affirmations while connecting with nature. By combining meditation, affirmations, and nature connection, we can foster a more harmonious relationship among our different personas and our authentic self.

Create a set of affirmations for each of your personas. During meditation, repeat these affirmations while connecting to nature, exploring how these identities can coexist harmoniously. Begin by writing affirmations that capture the positive aspects of each persona you've identified. For example, for a "nurturing parent" persona, you might write, "I am caring and supportive."

Find a quiet spot in nature for your meditation practice. As you sit comfortably, connect with your surroundings using your senses. Then, slowly repeat each affirmation, allowing yourself to feel the truth of the statement. Visualize how this aspect of yourself interacts with nature and your other personas. Notice any feelings of resistance or harmony that arise.

Repeat this process for 3–5 personas. After your meditation, reflect on how these different aspects of yourself can work together in harmony, both in nature and in your daily life.

Example: Lilah created affirmations for her "ambitious professional" and "free-spirited artist" personas. While meditating in a garden, she repeated, "I am driven and creative." She visualized these aspects working together, with nature inspiring her work and her ambition fueling her artistic pursuits. This practice helped Lilah integrate these seemingly conflicting parts of herself, leading to a more balanced approach to her career and hobbies.

Our Ever-Changing Roles

Former President of India A. P. J. Abdul Kalam once said, "We are all actors in a play, and the roles we take on reflect who we are at the moment." This quote reflects the fluid nature of identity and how we adapt our personas to different life circumstances. By examining the various social masks we wear, we can uncover truths about our identity and forge the opportunity to connect with our authentic selves.

Chapter Three

The Hidden Self

Embracing Your Shadow

When we venture into nature, we often seek peace, clarity, and connection. However, the wilderness can also serve as a mirror, reflecting aspects of ourselves we may overlook or deny. These hidden parts, our "shadow," hold the key to deeper self-awareness and personal growth. By acknowledging and integrating these concealed elements of our psyche, we can become more conscious, authentic, and whole.

Nature provides an ideal backdrop for inner exploration, offering a space free from everyday distractions and societal expectations. As you immerse yourself in the natural world, you may find that your Shadow emerges more readily, presenting opportunities for profound self-discovery and transformation. Embracing your Shadow in nature can lead to a more genuine connection with yourself, others, and the environment around you.

The Cave of Echoes

In an ancient land, a deep cave known as the Cave of Echoes was feared by the villagers for generations. It was said that those who entered would confront their deepest fears. One day, a brave young woman named Mira, feeling burdened by her emotions, decided to venture into the cave.

As she stepped inside, the walls whispered echoes of her doubts, insecurities, and past traumas. Overwhelmed, she felt compelled to flee. But then, she remembered the stories of old—how the shadows held the key to self-discovery. Instead of running, Mira sat amidst the darkness, confronting each shadow that emerged. One by one, she acknowledged her fears as parts of her being rather than foes to battle. As she accepted them, the echoes transformed into gentle whispers of wisdom. By the time she emerged from the cave, Mira carried not just the weight of her past but the light of understanding, infusing her with newfound strength and empowerment.

Reflection

This story illustrates the importance of confronting one's shadow. Nature can provide a metaphorical—or physical—cave that reveals our fears, teaching us that acknowledgment and acceptance of our hidden parts are essential for personal growth.

Exercises

1. Shadow Box in Nature

This exercise helps us externalize and confront hidden thoughts and emotions while being present in a natural environment, allowing for deeper self-reflection and awareness.

Find a small box or container. As you prepare to venture into nature, take a moment to sit quietly and reflect on any thoughts, feelings, or behaviors you typically push away or deny. Write each of these on separate, small slips of paper—but don't put them in the box yet. As you write, allow yourself to be honest and vulnerable, acknowledging aspects of yourself that you may find uncomfortable or challenging.

Once you're in nature, find a peaceful spot to sit. Take out your box and the slips of paper. Hold each slip, read its contents aloud, and place it in the box. As you do this, imagine you're creating a safe space for these hidden parts of yourself. When you're finished, close the box and set it aside.

Spend 15–20 more minutes allowing yourself to be present with your surroundings. Notice how you feel after acknowledging these shadow aspects. Then, open the box and review your slips. Look for patterns or recurring themes. Ask yourself: What needs or desires might these shadow aspects be trying to express? How can I integrate these parts of myself more fully?

As you prepare to leave, decide which slips to keep in the box and which to release. For those you keep, commit to working on integrating these aspects. For those you release, find a natural way to dispose of them: bury them, let them float down a stream, or scatter them in the wind. This symbolic act represents your willingness to acknowledge and transform these parts of yourself.

Continue this practice regularly, adding new slips as you become aware of other shadow aspects. Over time, you may notice a shift in your self-awareness and a greater sense of wholeness.

Example: Willa, an environmental activist, used the shadow box exercise during a weekend camping trip. She wrote down feelings of anger towards those who seemed indifferent to climate change. Through this process, she recognized her own moments of environmental carelessness and found ways to approach her activism with more compassion and understanding.

2. Shadow Collage

This visual exercise helps us explore and integrate contrasting aspects of our personality, fostering greater self-awareness and reducing internal conflict.

Before heading into nature, gather magazines, newspapers, or printed images, along with scissors, glue, and a large piece of paper or cardboard. Once in a natural setting, find a quiet, comfortable spot to work where you won't be disturbed.

Begin by reflecting on the different personas or roles you embody in your life. Consider both the aspects you readily show to the world and those you tend to hide or suppress. As you flip through the images, intuitively select those that resonate with these various aspects of yourself. Don't overthink your choices; let your subconscious guide you.

Divide your paper or cardboard into two sections. On one side, arrange and glue images representing your "public" self—the qualities and behaviors you're comfortable displaying to others—in a way that feels meaningful to you. On the other side, place images that represent your shadow self—the traits, desires, or emotions you typically keep hidden.

As you create your collage, pay attention to your thoughts and feelings. Notice any resistance or discomfort that arises as you acknowledge your shadow aspects. Take breaks to observe nature around you, allowing its

presence to ground and support you in this process.

Once your collage is complete, spend time observing it as a whole. Notice the contrasts and connections between your public and shadow selves. Reflect on how these different aspects might be creating tension or

stress in your life. Ask yourself: How can I integrate these contrasting parts more harmoniously? What strengths or gifts might my shadow self be offering? In your journal, write down any insights or realizations that arose from this exercise. Consider how you might bring more balance to your life by acknowledging and embracing your shadow aspects.

Keep your collage as a visual reminder of your inner landscape. Revisit it periodically, especially when facing challenges or making important decisions. Use it as a tool to check in with yourself and ensure you're honoring all aspects of your being.

Example: Nathan, a corporate executive, created a shadow collage during a solo hiking trip. His public side showed images of success and control, while his shadow side revealed a desire for creativity and spontaneity. This insight led him to incorporate more artistic pursuits into his life, bringing greater balance and fulfillment.

3. Shadow Sitting

This meditative practice helps us connect with and acknowledge hidden aspects of ourselves while remaining grounded in our natural environment, fostering greater self-acceptance and reducing stress.

Find a quiet, secluded spot in nature where you feel safe and comfortable. Sit in a relaxed position, either on the ground or on a natural surface like a rock or fallen log. Begin by closing your eyes and taking several deep breaths, allowing yourself to settle into the present moment. As you breathe deeply, imagine you're creating a protective circle of light around yourself. This circle represents a safe space where all parts of you are welcome and accepted.

Gradually shift your attention inward, becoming aware of your thoughts, emotions, and bodily sensations. Invite your shadow—those parts of yourself you typically avoid or deny—to join you in this circle. As you do this, you may notice certain thoughts, emotions, or memories arising. Welcome them without judgment, simply observing their presence.

If you encounter resistance or discomfort, acknowledge it gently. Remind yourself that this is a safe space for exploration and that all aspects of yourself are worthy of attention and acceptance.

As you sit with your shadow, ask it what it needs from you. Listen intently, allowing any insights or messages to come through. You might receive these as words, images, or sensations in your body; trust whatever arises. If strong emotions surface, allow yourself to feel them fully while staying grounded in your physical presence in nature. Let the steadiness of the earth beneath you and the rhythm of your breath anchor you.

As you conclude the meditation, express gratitude to your shadow for its presence and any insights it has shared. Gradually bring your awareness back to your surroundings, noticing the sounds, smells, and textures of nature around you.

Take a few moments to journal about your experience. Write down any revelations, emotions, or questions that arose during the meditation. Consider how you might integrate these shadow aspects more fully into your daily life.

Practice shadow sitting regularly, allowing nature to support you in this deep inner work. Over time, you may notice a greater sense of self-acceptance, reduced stress, and a more authentic way of being in the world.

Example: Christina, a therapist, practiced shadow sitting during a retreat in the mountains. She encountered her fear of vulnerability, realizing how it affected her relationships. This awareness led her to open up more with loved ones and clients, deepening her connections and enhancing her professional work.

The Power to Change

Writer–philanthropist Sheryl Sandberg once said, "We cannot change what we are not aware of, and once we are aware, we cannot help but change." This quote highlights the importance of self-awareness in personal transformation. By confronting our shadow and integrating hidden aspects of ourselves into our identity, we can foster growth and a foundation of authenticity.

Chapter Four

Archetypes as Guides

Archetypes, universal symbols and patterns deeply ingrained in human consciousness, offer a powerful lens through which we can explore our relationship with nature and ourselves. By recognizing and engaging with these primordial images in natural settings, we can unlock deeper levels of self-awareness. As we immerse ourselves in the natural world, archetypes emerge, reflecting aspects of our psyche and guiding us towards a more profound understanding of our place within the greater tapestry of life.

The Weaver of Stories

In a vibrant meadow, there lived a storyteller named Prior, skilled in weaving tales that reflected ancient archetypes. The meadow itself was a tapestry of characters—the Wise Old Man, the Nurturing Mother, and the Courageous Hero. One day, a curious child approached Prior, seeking to understand his own life story.

The child wandered into the meadow and encountered each archetype in its natural state. The Wise Old Man shared insights about patience, the Nurturing Mother taught the value of empathy, and the Courageous Hero sparked the spirit of adventure within him.

Returning to Prior, the child realized that he contained all these archetypes within him. He thanked Prior for guiding him to this awakening, recognizing that understanding these roles enriched his identity.

Reflection

This myth emphasizes the value of archetypes in our lives. Nature often embodies these archetypes, allowing individuals to explore varied aspects of themselves, fostering self-awareness and a sense of belonging.

Exercises

1. Archetype Observation Exercise

This exercise is designed to help us identify and connect with archetypal energies present in different natural environments. By observing which archetypes emerge in various settings, we can gain insights into how these universal patterns influence our experience of nature and our own psyche. This practice enhances self-awareness by revealing the interplay between our inner world and the natural world around us.

Spend time in various natural settings (e.g., in a forest, at the beach, near a mountain) and observe which archetypes emerge from those environments (e.g., the Sage in the mountains, the Nurturer by the water). Note your reflections on how these archetypes influence your experience in nature.

Example: During a recent hike in the mountains, Delia felt the presence of the Sage archetype. The towering peaks and vast vistas inspired a sense of wisdom and perspective, and she found herself contemplating life's bigger questions and feeling a deep connection to ancient knowledge. This experience helped Delia tap into her own inner wisdom and approach challenges with a broader, more philosophical outlook.

2. Archetypal Traits List

This exercise helps us identify and explore the archetypes that resonate most strongly with us. By examining the traits, strengths, and challenges associated with these archetypes, we can gain a deeper understanding of our own personality and behavior patterns. This self-reflection can lead to greater self-awareness and provide insights into how we interact with nature and the world around us.

Write a list of three to five archetypes you resonate with most. For each archetype, include traits, strengths, and challenges, and reflect on how these characteristics influence your actions and choices in natural settings.

Example: While doing the archetypal traits exercise, Randall resonated strongly with the Explorer archetype. Randall listed some of the traits of this archetype (curiosity, adventurousness, and independence) as well as some of the strengths (adaptability and openness to new experiences). However, he noted that challenges involved restlessness and difficulty committing. In nature, this archetype drove Randall to seek out hidden trails and unexplored areas, pushing him beyond his comfort zone and fostering personal growth through new and challenging experiences.

3. Archetype Movement Exploration

This exercise encourages us to embody different archetypal energies through movement in a natural setting. By physically expressing these universal patterns, we can deepen our connection to both the archetypes and the natural world. This practice enhances body awareness, promotes mindfulness, and offers a unique way to explore how different archetypal energies influence our experience of nature and ourselves.

Choose a different archetype each day and develop a movement practice that embodies its qualities. Take this practice outdoors, engaging in it for 15–20 minutes, and observe how this archetypal energy influences your body and spirit.

Example: During this exercise, Mona embodied the Warrior archetype during her morning walk in the park. She focused on strong, purposeful movements, maintaining an upright posture and taking decisive steps. As she moved, she felt a surge of confidence and determination. The Warrior energy helped Mona face the day's challenges with courage and resolve, reminding her of her inner strength and resilience in the face of adversity.

Learning From Myths

American writer Joseph Campbell wrote, "Myth is the greatest of all teachers." This quote underscores the value of myths and archetypes in guiding self-discovery and personal growth. By exploring archetypes in nature as reflections of our own psyche, we can discover pathways to deeper understanding.

Chapter Five

Embracing Duality
The Masculine & Feminine

The interplay of masculine and feminine energies within nature offers a profound pathway to personal growth. By recognizing and embracing these complementary forces, we can gain deeper insights into our own inner landscapes. This exploration allows us to become more conscious of our thoughts, emotions, and actions, fostering a harmonious balance within ourselves and our environment.

The Dance of the Elements

In a land where the sun kissed the earth each day, two ancient spirits reigned: Solaris, the solar spirit representing masculine strength, and Luna, the luminous spirit embodying feminine grace. They danced a timeless dance of balance, their energies creating the harmony of seasons.

However, one year, Solaris became overzealous, radiating excessive heat and draining life from the earth. Sensing the imbalance, Luna gently approached him, urging to restore harmony. Together, they invoked the equinox, creating a beautiful convergence of energies where day and night became equal.

As the earth thrived once more, each understood that their energies complemented one another. Through their dance, they taught the world the importance of nurturing both strength and compassion.

Reflection

This story illustrates the need for balance between the masculine and feminine energies within ourselves and within nature. Recognizing and honoring both energies fosters self-awareness, enriching our experience and understanding of the world.

Exercises

1. Energy Exploration in Nature

This exercise invites us to consciously embody first masculine then feminine energy during a day spent in nature. By intentionally focusing on one energy at a time, we'll gain a deeper understanding of how each energy influences our perceptions, actions, and feelings. This heightened awareness can lead to valuable insights about our own tendencies and areas for growth.

Choose a day to spend in nature, deciding beforehand whether you'll embody masculine or feminine energy. If focusing on masculine energy, emphasize traits like assertiveness, goal-oriented thinking, and analytical observation. For feminine energy, concentrate on receptivity, intuition, and emotional connection.

As you explore your surroundings, pay attention to how this energy focus affects your experience of the environment, your interactions with others, and your internal state. Notice any shifts in your perception, decision making, or emotional responses. At the end of the day, reflect on what you learned about yourself and how this experience can inform your daily life.

The next day, choose to embody the other energy and conduct the same exercise. Notice the difference in how you feel and what behaviors you engage in when embodying this energy versus the other.

Example: Devon chose to embody feminine energy during a hike. He found himself more attuned to the subtle sounds of the forest and felt a deep emotional connection to the landscape. This experience helped him recognize the value of slowing down and being more receptive in his daily life, balancing his usually assertive approach to challenges.

2. Partnered Nature Walk

This exercise encourages us to explore the balance of masculine and feminine energies through dialogue and shared experience in nature. By discussing these concepts with a partner while immersed in the natural world, we can gain new perspectives on how these energies manifest in our life and environment.

Invite a friend or partner for a nature walk. As you explore, discuss your understanding of masculine and feminine energies and how you see them reflected in the environment around you. Take turns pointing out examples of each energy in nature, such as the protective strength of a large tree (masculine) or the nurturing quality of a flowing stream (feminine). Reflect on how these energies manifest in your own lives and relationships. Consider how you might bring more balance to areas where one energy dominates.

As you walk, consciously try to embody a balance of both energies, noticing how this affects your interaction with nature and each other.

Example: Mark and Phil's nature walk led to a profound discussion about their friendship dynamics. They realized that Mark often took on a nurturing role (feminine energy), while Phil tended to be more assertive (masculine energy) in their social life. This awareness helped them appreciate their complementary strengths and inspired them to cultivate more balance in their interactions.

3. Poetry of Duality

This creative exercise encourages us to express the interplay of masculine and feminine energies through poetry inspired by nature. By using natural imagery as metaphors for these energies, we'll deepen our understanding of their presence in both the external world and our inner self.

Find a quiet, comfortable spot in nature to observe and reflect. As you take in your surroundings, note elements that embody masculine energy (e.g., a tall mountain, a thunderstorm) and feminine energy (e.g., a calm lake, a blooming flower). Use these observations as inspiration to write a poem that explores the balance and interplay of these energies. Consider how these natural elements mirror aspects of your own personality or life experiences.

Craft a short poem using your observations, reflecting also on how embracing both energies might lead to greater wholeness and self-awareness. After writing, read your poem aloud, allowing its message to resonate within you and your surroundings.

Example: Jen's poem contrasted the sturdy oak (masculine) with the flowing river (feminine). As she wrote, she realized how her own life mirrored this duality: her career ambitions represented the oak's strength, while her emotional support for friends reflected the river's nurturing flow. This insight inspired Jen cultivate more balance between her personal and professional life.

Harnessing the Energies Within Us

Author Marianne Williamson once wrote, "We need to stop diverting the power of our feminine energy into criticism and judgment and instead learn to work together." This quote emphasizes the need for balance and cooperation between masculine and feminine energies. By embracing both aspects, we can work toward personal growth and harmonious relationships with ourselves and with nature.

Chapter Six

Harnessing Active Imagination

A ctive imagination serves as a powerful tool for deepening our connection with nature and ourselves. By engaging our creative faculties while immersed in natural settings, we open doorways to enhanced self-awareness. This practice allows us to tap into the wisdom of our inner world, using nature as a canvas for exploration and reflection. Through active imagination, we can uncover hidden aspects of our psyche, confront challenges, and cultivate a more profound sense of unity with the world around us.

The Garden of Dreams

In a hidden valley, a young girl named Eden discovered a lush garden that transformed with the seasons. Each night, as she slept nearby, she wandered into this garden through her dreams, unlocking the door to her imagination.

One night, while exploring the garden, she encountered talking flowers, each sharing a piece of wisdom from her subconscious. The daisies spoke of simplicity, the roses conveyed love, and the thorns reminded her of the challenges she's experienced. Each element reflected her inner world, showcasing aspects of herself she had yet to explore.

By immersing herself in this active imagination, Eden began to realize how her inner garden mirrored her thoughts and feelings. This awareness allowed her to cultivate her emotions mindfully, shaping her reality with intention.

Reflection

This tale illustrates how engaging in active imagination can help us connect with the different facets of ourselves. Nature can serve as a powerful backdrop for inner exploration, leading to authentic self-awareness and understanding.

Exercises

1. Imagined Nature Encounter

This exercise harnesses the power of visualization and dialogue to deepen our connection with nature and our inner selves. By imaginatively engaging with a natural element, we can access insights about our emotions, challenges, and personal growth.

Find a quiet, comfortable space where you won't be disturbed. Begin by closing your eyes and taking several deep breaths, allowing yourself to relax and become centered. Now, visualize yourself in a natural setting, focusing on a specific element like a tree, rock, or river. Imagine this element coming to life and engaging you in conversation. What does it say? What questions do you ask in return? Pay attention to the insights, emotions, and revelations that arise during this dialogue.

Continue the conversation until it comes to a natural close. Then, slowly open your eyes and journal about your experience, reflecting on what you learned about yourself and your connection to nature.

Example: Rachel, a busy executive, practiced this exercise and visualized a conversation with an old oak tree. The tree spoke of patience and deep roots, helping her realize her need for stability and long-term planning in her career. This insight led her to re-evaluate her work-life balance and make changes that aligned more closely with her goals.

2. Dream Imagery Exploration

This exercise taps into the rich symbolism of our dreams, particularly those featuring natural elements, to uncover deeper layers of self-awareness. By recording and reflecting on these dreams, we can bridge the gap between our unconscious mind and our waking experiences in nature.

Keep a dream journal by your bedside. Upon waking, immediately write down any dreams you remember, paying special attention to those featuring natural elements or settings. Note the vivid imagery, characters, and emotions present in the dream.

Later, reflect on these elements and how they might connect to your waking life, personal challenges, or relationship with nature. Consider how you might engage with these dream symbols in your daily life or during time spent in nature. Look for patterns or recurring themes in your dreams over time.

Example: Channing consistently dreamed of a mountain he couldn't climb. After reflecting on this imagery, he realized it represented his fear of career advancement in many areas of life. This awareness prompted him to seek new challenges at work and start hiking on weekends, gradually building his confidence both professionally and in his connection with nature.

3. Body Storytelling

This exercise integrates physical movement with imaginative exploration, allowing us to express our inner world while immersed in nature. By physically enacting our internal characters and feelings, we can gain new insights and foster a deeper connection between our inner and outer experiences.

Choose a natural setting where you feel comfortable moving freely. Begin by closing your eyes and taking several deep breaths to center yourself. Now, tune into your inner world, identifying a character, emotion, or aspect of yourself you'd like to explore. Next, open your eyes and begin to move through the natural space, allowing your body to fully embody and express this inner element. Use gestures, postures, and movements that feel authentic to this part of you.

As you move, be aware of how your body interacts with the natural environment around you. Continue this practice for 15–20 minutes. When you're finished, take some time to reflect on your experience, noting any insights or emotions that arose.

Example: Hannah, struggling with self-doubt, embodied her inner critic while walking through a forest. As she moved, she noticed her posture becoming hunched and her steps hesitant. Gradually, she allowed her movements to become more open and fluid, mirroring the trees around her. This physical exploration helped Lisa recognize and release some of her self-limiting beliefs, fostering a new sense of confidence and connection with nature.

The Power of Imagination

Albert Einstein once said, "Imagination is more important than knowledge—for knowledge is limited, whereas imagination embraces the entire world, stimulating progress, giving birth to evolution." Einstein's words highlight the power of imagination in fostering creativity and personal evolution. Using active imagination as a tool for self-discovery and connection to nature, we can work toward true authenticity in our lives and relationships.

Chapter Seven

Alchemical Transformation

Alchemy, often misunderstood as the mere pursuit of turning base metals into gold, is a profound metaphor for personal transformation. When applied to our experiences in nature, it becomes a powerful tool for self-discovery and growth. By viewing our interactions with the natural world through an alchemical lens, we can unlock deeper levels of consciousness and self-awareness. This process invites us to see the parallels between nature's transformative cycles and our own inner evolution, fostering a sense of connection and purpose that transcends our everyday existence.

The Potion of Transformation

In a mystical forest, an ancient alchemist named Zephyr sought to create the ultimate potion of transformation. He believed that deep within the forest lay unique ingredients that held the secrets to self-discovery.

One day, on a journey, Zephyr gathered petals, leaves, and crystals. With each element, he reflected on its significance—strength, healing, and wisdom. As he combined these ingredients in his cauldron, he understood that true transformation must begin within.

As the potion bubbled, a vision emerged—showing him a path of self-acceptance and the merging of his talents. The alchemical process taught him that by mixing the elements of his life, he could discover his true self and create his own identity.

Reflection

This myth illustrates the alchemical process of transformation—the journey through personal experiences—can lead to growth and realization. Engaging with nature allows us to discover elements within themselves that are crucial for authentic transformation.

Exercises

1. Alchemical Symbols Exploration

This exercise is designed to deepen our understanding of alchemical symbolism and its relevance to our personal growth journey. By researching and creatively interpreting alchemical symbols, we'll forge a personal connection to these ancient concepts, enhancing our self-awareness and providing a visual framework for our transformative experiences in nature.

Begin by researching common alchemical symbols such as the Philosopher's Stone, the Four Elements (i.e., Earth, Water, Air, Fire), the Ouroboros, and the stages of the Great Work (i.e., Nigredo, Albedo, Citrinitas, Rubedo). Select three to five of these symbols that resonate with you personally and create a visual representation or collage that incorporates them. This can be a drawing, painting, digital artwork, or a physical collage using found objects and images.

As you create, reflect on why each symbol speaks to you and how it relates to your experiences in nature. Write brief notes explaining your personal interpretation of each symbol and how it connects to your journey of self-discovery.

Example: Eve, an avid hiker, chose the symbols of the Four Elements and the Ouroboros for her collage. She used pressed leaves and soil to represent Earth, a blue watercolor wash for Water, feathers for Air, and red and orange tissue paper for Fire. The Ouroboros, a serpent eating its own tail, encircled these elements, symbolizing the cyclical nature of growth she experienced on her wilderness treks. This visual representation helped Eve understand how each element of nature contributed to her ongoing personal transformation.

2. Nature's Transformative Elements

This exercise encourages us to observe and reflect on the transformative processes in nature, drawing parallels to our own personal growth. By mindfully engaging with natural cycles and changes, we can develop a deeper understanding of our own capacity for transformation and the interconnectedness of all living things.

Choose a natural setting you can visit regularly over a period of time (e.g., a local park, your backyard, or a nearby forest). Commit to observing this space at least once a week for a month or longer. During each visit, focus on identifying and documenting natural transformations. This could include seasonal changes, plant growth cycles, weather patterns, or animal behaviors.

Keep a journal of your observations, noting both the physical changes you see and your emotional responses to them. After each visit, reflect on how these natural transformations mirror your own experiences of growth or change. Consider the following questions:

- How does the resilience and adaptability of nature inspire me?

- What personal transformations am I currently experiencing?

- How can I apply nature's wisdom to my own life?

Example: Carlos visited a local pond weekly for two months. He observed tadpoles transforming into frogs, noting their gradual changes. This process resonated with his own slow but steady progress in overcoming social anxiety. Carlos realized that, like the tadpoles, his transformation required patience and the right environment. He found comfort in nature's rhythm, understanding that personal growth, like the frog's metamorphosis, unfolds in its own time.

3. Elemental Alchemy Reflection

This meditative exercise helps us connect with the four alchemical elements (Earth, Water, Air, Fire) in a natural setting. By focusing on these elemental forces and their transformative qualities, we'll gain insights into our own alchemical process of personal growth and self-discovery.

Find a quiet, natural setting where you feel safe and comfortable. Sit or lie down in a relaxed position and begin with several deep breaths to center yourself. Next, focus your attention on each of the four elements in turn, spending about 5–10 minutes with each:

- *Earth*: Feel the solid ground beneath you. Reflect on stability, grounding, and material manifestation in your life.

- *Water*: Listen for any water sounds or imagine a flowing stream. Consider fluidity, emotions, and adaptability in your journey.

- *Air*: Feel the breeze on your skin or observe the movement of leaves. Contemplate mental clarity, communication, and new ideas.

- *Fire*: Feel the warmth of the sun or visualize a flame. Reflect on transformation, passion, and energy in your personal growth.

As you connect with each element, consider how its qualities can assist you in your own personal alchemical process. What aspects of your life need more stability (Earth), fluidity (Water), clarity (Air), or transformation (Fire)? After meditating on all four elements, take some time to journal about your insights and any actions you feel inspired to take.

Example: During her elemental meditation, Riley realized she had been neglecting her need for stability (Earth) in pursuit of constant change. The gentle persistence of a nearby stream (Water) inspired her to approach her goals with steady, adaptable effort rather than forceful bursts. The breeze (Air) cleared her mind, helping her articulate a new career direction. The sun's warmth (Fire) ignited her passion to take decisive action. This elemental reflection helped Riley balance and align her approach to personal growth.

Be The Change

Gandhi famously said, "You must be the change you wish to see in the world." This quote calls for personal responsibility in self-transformation, encouraging us to engage with nature to become the best versions of ourselves.

Chapter Eight

Awakening Through Synchronicity

I n the hustle of modern life, we often overlook the subtle messages nature provides. Synchronicity—those meaningful coincidences that seem to guide us—can serve as a bridge between our inner world and the natural environment. By attuning ourselves to these moments, we can cultivate a deeper sense of self-awareness and connection to the world around us. This practice not only enhances our personal growth but also fosters a more profound respect for the environment and our place within it.

The Trail of Whispers

In a picturesque landscape, there lived an elder named Selene who believed deeply in the magic of synchronicity. One afternoon, while walking along a familiar path, she noticed a series of peculiar coincidences: a butterfly landing on her shoulder, a flower blooming as she paused, and a robin singing from a nearby tree.

Awed by these experiences, she decided to follow the butterfly, feeling guided to uncover deeper meanings. Each step led her to a gathering of creatures all sharing stories, each resonating with the signs she had previously encountered.

As the creatures communicated, Selene recognized that these synchronicities were a tapestry of connection, all leading to this moment of gathering and unity in nature. She returned home filled with gratitude, understanding that the universe has the power to guide us subtly through signs.

Reflection

This story illustrates the concept of synchronicity—the meaningful coincidences we experience that can guide us toward and through self-discovery. Nature often provides the context through which we find connections, leading to greater awareness of our journey.

Exercises

1. Messages from Nature

This exercise is designed to heighten our awareness of the natural world and its potential to offer insights into our inner life. By actively engaging with nature and noting significant signs or symbols, we can develop a deeper connection with our environment and uncover meaningful parallels to our personal experiences.

Spend time in a natural setting, noting any signs or symbols that stand out to you, such as an unusual cloud shape or a specific bird call. Reflect on how these messages might relate to your current life situation or thoughts.

Example: During a walk in the park, Lawrence noticed a persistent robin following his path. As he contemplated a career change, the bird's presence reminded him of the saying "a little bird told me." This synchronicity encouraged Lawrence to trust his instincts about pursuing a new job opportunity, ultimately leading him to a fulfilling career shift that aligned with his passions.

2. Inspirational Poetry

Poetry has long been a medium for expressing profound truths and connecting with the deeper aspects of the human experience. This exercise encourages us to tap into our creative side while exploring the concept of synchronicity in nature. By crafting a poem, we'll engage both our analytical and intuitive mind, potentially uncovering new insights about our relationship with the natural world and our own emotional landscape.

Write a poem that captures the essence of synchronicity and its relationship with nature, as you see it. Use metaphors and imagery that highlight the intertwining of human experiences—especially your own—with the natural world.

Example: Ann, an aspiring poet, wrote about a fallen leaf that landed on her notebook while she pondered life changes. The poem explored themes of letting go and new beginnings, mirroring the leaf's journey. This creative process helped Ann process her emotions about a recent breakup and find solace in nature's cycles of renewal.

3. Synchronicity Celebration Ritual

Rituals can be powerful tools for reinforcing positive experiences and integrating them into our lives. This exercise invites us to create a personal ritual to honor moments of synchronicity, using natural elements as symbols. By doing so, we can cultivate gratitude for these meaningful coincidences and strengthen our connection to both nature and our inner wisdom.

Create a personal ritual to celebrate moments of synchronicity. Use natural items (e.g., stones, feathers) to symbolize these experiences and express gratitude for the connections they represent in your life.

Example: Julia created a small altar in her garden where she placed a unique stone for each significant synchronicity she had experienced recently. During her weekly ritual, she would hold each stone, recalling the associated event and expressing gratitude. This practice helped Julia maintain a positive outlook and increased her awareness of meaningful coincidences in her daily life.

Synchronicities All Around Us

Carl Jung said, "Synchronicity is an ever-present reality for those who have eyes to see." This quote speaks to the significance of recognizing meaningful coincidences in our lives. Through exploring synchronicities in nature, we can enhance our self-awareness and guide ourselves toward personal growth.

Chapter Nine

Nurturing Your Authentic Self

A Path to Greater Consciousness

The concept of "the self" offers a profound pathway to heightened consciousness, particularly when immersed in nature. By engaging with the natural world, we can tap into a deeper understanding of our true essence, transcending societal roles and expectations. Nature provides a mirror for our inner landscape, allowing us to reflect on our authentic selves and foster personal growth. This journey of self-discovery in nature's embrace can lead to a more fulfilling and conscious way of living.

The Journey to the Heartwood

In a great enchanted forest, a wandering seeker named Faelan embarked on a journey to find the Heartwood Tree, said to hold the essence of the Self. In his adventures, he encountered various beings—the wise old turtle, the playful fox, and the majestic eagle, each representing different aspects of his character.

As he traveled, Faelan faced challenges that called forth his courage, creativity, and intuition. With each encounter, he began to merge these qualities into a cohesive understanding of himself. Finally, after what seemed like an exhausting quest, he stood before the Heartwood Tree, large and majestic, radiating a soft glow.

Realizing that the tree was not separate from him, but rather a representation of all the experiences he had gathered along the way, Faelan embraced the full spectrum of his being. In that moment, he felt whole.

Reflection

This story underscores how the journey toward the self—the process of individuation—nurtures self-awareness and understanding. Nature plays a crucial role in leading us to discover our multifaceted identities, ultimately promising wholeness and integration.

Exercises

1. Nature Contemplation Exercise

This exercise encourages deep reflection in a natural environment, helping us shed societal labels and connect with our core self. By immersing ourselves in nature's tranquility, we create space for authentic self-discovery and increased awareness.

Find a serene, beautiful spot in nature, like a forest clearing, a quiet beach, or a mountain overlook. Sit comfortably and take several deep breaths, allowing yourself to relax and become present.

As you observe your surroundings, begin to contemplate your true essence. Ask yourself: Who am I beyond my job, relationships, and social roles? What qualities define my authentic self? Allow nature's rhythms and beauty to guide your introspection and bring you clarity. Notice any insights or emotions that arise, accepting them without judgment. Spend at least 30 minutes in this contemplative state, allowing nature to mirror your inner landscape.

Example: Fred, a busy executive, spent an afternoon by a serene lake. As he watched the ripples on the water, he realized his constant striving for success had overshadowed his true passions. The peaceful setting helped him reconnect with his love for art and his desire to create. This insight led Fred to incorporate more creativity into his life, bringing greater fulfillment and balance.

2. Self-Discovery Ceremony

This ceremony creates a sacred space for acknowledging and celebrating our journey of self-discovery. By incorporating natural elements as symbols, we deepen our connection to both nature and our authentic self, fostering greater self-awareness and personal growth.

Choose a meaningful outdoor location for your ceremony. Gather natural objects that resonate with different aspects of your identity—perhaps a stone for strength, a leaf for growth, or a feather for freedom. Create a small altar or circle with these items.

Begin the ceremony by grounding yourself through deep breathing or meditation. Then, pick up each object one by one, reflecting on the aspect of yourself it represents. As you hold each item, consider how it relates to your true self and your journey of self-discovery. Express gratitude for each quality and the insights you've gained. Conclude the ceremony by making a commitment to continue your path of self-awareness and growth.

Example: Henry conducted his ceremony on a hilltop at sunset. He used a pinecone to represent resilience, recalling how he'd overcome personal challenges. A smooth river stone symbolized inner peace, reminding him of the calm he'd cultivated through meditation. This ritual helped Henry integrate various aspects of his identity, leading to a more holistic self-understanding and renewed commitment to personal growth.

3. Mentorship in Self-Exploration

This exercise allows us to share our insights and experiences while supporting another person's growth. By guiding someone through nature-based self-exploration, we deepen our own understanding of the self while fostering greater consciousness in others.

Acting as a mentor, guide choose a friend or family member to guide on their journey of self-discovery, encouraging them to engage with nature along the way. Help them uncover connections between their experiences in the natural world and their understanding of the self. Begin by discussing the concept of the self with your mentee, emphasizing the role of nature in self-discovery. Plan a series of nature outings together, choosing diverse environments like forests, beaches, or mountains.

During these excursions, encourage your mentee to observe their thoughts, feelings, and reactions to the natural surroundings. Guide them in drawing parallels between nature's processes and their own life journey. Ask open-ended questions to prompt reflection, such as "How does this landscape reflect your inner world?" or "What qualities in nature resonate with your true self?" After each outing, discuss insights gained and how they relate to self-awareness and personal growth.

Example: Phoebe mentored her colleague, James, in self-exploration through nature. During a hike, she encouraged James to observe a stream's journey, relating it to his own life path. This metaphor helped James recognize his resilience in navigating obstacles. Their discussions after each outing deepened James's self-awareness, while Phoebe gained new perspectives on her own journey through the mentoring process.

The Essence of Being

Indian guru Sadhguru said, "To know oneself, one must know the essence of being." This quote emphasizes the importance of self-discovery as a path to understanding our true nature. Connecting with our authentic self through nature can fostering greater consciousness and self-awareness.

Chapter Ten

What's New?

Congratulations on completing your journey through Nature's Wisdom. You've taken an important step in your journey guided by nature by exploring the complexities of the self and your relationship with others and the world around you. Each chapter has provided you with unique insights and practical exercises designed to empower you to attune yourself to the natural world and nurture your own well-being. As you reflect on your experiences, consider the following action steps to integrate your newfound knowledge into your everyday life:

Reflect on Your Growth:

Take some time to revisit the sections of this book that resonated with you the most. Reflect on what you've learned about yourself, the environment, and your relationship with the natural world. Create a routine that includes journaling, meditating, or both to foster deep reflection and capture your insights and emotions. Engage in this self-reflection regularly; it will help you maintain awareness as you navigate future challenges.

Set Intentions for the Future:

As you move forward, take a moment to envision your desired future. What aspirations do you have for the coming weeks, months, and years related to your connection with nature? Write down these intentions, and revisit them regularly, allowing them to guide your actions and decisions. Setting clear goals for your personal evolution as you continue your journey will help you remain aligned with your authentic self.

Engage in Mindfulness:

Maintain a mindful approach to your daily life. Practice being present and aware of your surroundings, your thoughts, and feelings. Regular practices such as meditation, journaling, or mindful observation of nature, can help you remain centered and present. These practices will support you in staying connected to your emotions without becoming overwhelmed.

Integrate Learnings into Your Daily Life:

Make a conscious effort to incorporate the lessons and values you've learned here into your daily life and connection with nature. Create and commit to a regular routine that incorporates these practices and allow them to evolve as you continue to process your emotions and experiences.

Practice Self-Care & -Compassion:

Remember to always be gentle and compassionate with yourself as you continue to journey through life with the help of nature's wisdom. Healing is not linear: growth takes time, and it's okay to experience setbacks. Practice kindness towards yourself in these moments, recognizing your strengths and celebrating your journey. Develop a daily practice that nurtures you, whether through self-care routines, hobbies that bring you joy, or spending time with supportive friends and family. Your well-being, both mental and physical, is essential for you to navigate life's challenges and opportunities.

Honor Your Progress:

Just by completing this book, you have made significant strides. Celebrate the growth you've achieved throughout this process. Acknowledge both the small victories and the significant transformations. This gratitude will reinforce your journey and empower you as you step into your next chapter.

Connect With Your Community:

Engaging with community can provide encouragement, understanding, and opportunities for shared growth. Connect with others who are on a similar journey and share your experiences, insights, and challenges. Seek support from loved ones or find a forum or workshop where you can engage in discussions about nature as you continue to heal and grow. Remember, you're not alone on this journey. Your story has the potential to inspire and uplift, creating a ripple effect of awareness and understanding.

Remain Open & Continue Learning

Life will continue to unfold, and with it, new challenges and opportunities. Stay open to new experiences and commit to continuously learning about yourself and your relationship with the world around you. Embrace the unknown with curiosity and courage, knowing that every obstacle is an opportunity for further growth. Expanding your knowledge and experiences will empower you and those you love!

As you conclude this chapter and step into the next phase of your journey, remember to continue to tune into the world around you. By applying the principles you've learned and the tools you've developed throughout this book, you are equipped to navigate the challenges ahead with resilience and compassion. By committing to these practices and engaging with both nature and your inner self, you can cultivate a life rich in authenticity, awareness, and connection. Your journey forward is bright, filled with endless possibilities for personal growth and a richer understanding of life's unfolding narrative.

The Wisdom Manuals Series

Books That Bring Awareness, Compassion & Insights Into Your Everyday Life

This book is part of my Wisdom Manuals series. This book series was inspired first and foremost by a wish to incorporate spiritual wisdom into our daily lives. We are here to learn—to become conscious and awake throughout our lives. I truly believe that the way to find happiness and purpose in life is to be aware of all aspects of ourselves.

The Wisdom Manual series focuses on two things:

Helping us become more conscious—which helps us make good decisions, build self-awareness, engage in social interaction, solve problems, be more creative and productive, and be happier and more fulfilled

Integrating wisdom and consciousness into what we already do daily

Since I was very young, I've had questions about life. Why are we here? What are we supposed to learn? What is this thing called "wisdom," anyway?

Over the years, I have read many books about these very topics. But still, I have struggled with connecting with a single spiritual practice or disciplines. In many ways, creativity has become my spiritual go-to;I have found that the best wisdom can be found in what you experience in your body and daily life.

As a foundation for this series, I've usedJung's theory of the individuation process. Carl Gustav Jung (1875–1961) was a Swiss psychiatrist and psychoanalyst who founded analytical psychology.

Jung believed that our minds have two main parts: the part we're aware of (our conscious) and the part we're unaware of (our unconscious). He thought that to grow as people, we must understand and bring together these different parts of ourselves.

Jung came up with an idea called the "individuation process"—a journey we take to become complete and well balanced. Here's what this journey involves:

Getting to know different parts of ourselves, including how we act in public, our hidden thoughts and feelings, and typical behavior patterns all humans share

Understanding our dreams and using our imagination to learn more about our unconscious mind

Finding a balance between different sides of our personality, like the masculine and feminine qualities we all have

Becoming more "whole" and understanding ourselves better, including facing our inner struggles and accepting the good and bad parts of who we are

Not to be "perfect," but rather to become more truly ourselves, understanding and accepting our differences.

In the following pages, I offer short explanations of the concepts I use in my books:

Ego

Your ego is your sense of self—how you think of yourself and how you actin the world. It's the part of your mind that helps you make decisions, interact with others, and create your identity. Your ego helps you understand who you are and how you fit into your environment.

Persona

Your persona is the mask you wear when you are around other people—the version of yourself that you show to the world. This can include how you behave at work, with friends, or even in family settings. While the persona helps you fit in and connect with others, it can sometimes hide your true feelings or thoughts.

Shadow

Your shadow represents the parts of yourself that you try to keep hidden. This could include feelings, traits, or thoughts that you don't want to acknowledge—such as anger, fear, or insecurity. Everyone has a shadow, and understanding it can help you grow. Recognizing your shadow helps you acceptall parts of yourself—both the good and the bad.

Archetypes

Archetypes are universal symbols or themes found in stories, myths, and dreams. They represent different aspects of human experience. Examples include the Hero, the Caregiver, and the Rebel. These archetypes can guide you and shape your behavior by showing you the roles you might play in your life and relationships.

Masculine/Feminine Qualities

Everyone has both masculine and feminine qualities, regardless of gender or sex. Masculine traits might include strength and assertiveness, while feminine traits might include nurturing and compassion. Understanding these qualities helps you find balance within yourself. Acknowledging both sides can create a healthier view of relationships and personal growth.

Active Imagination

Active imagination is a technique that involves using your imagination to explore your thoughts and feelings. It often includes visualizing conversations with parts of yourself or characters from your dreams. This practice helps you tap into your inner thoughts and feelings, leading to better self-understanding.

Alchemy

Alchemy (the process of turning metals into gold) related to the self is about transformation. In Jung's work, it symbolizes turning negative feelings(like fear or pain) into positive growth (like wisdom or strength). The process of alchemy represents your journey to change and heal by learning from your experiences.

Synchronicity

Synchronicity refers to the meaningful coincidences that happen in your life. These events may be connected even if they don't appear to have a cause-and-effect relationship. Recognizing these moments can help you understand your path and feel more connected to the world around you.

Self

The self is the complete picture of who you are. It includes both your conscious and unconscious parts. Finding a balance between these aspects can lead to personal fulfillment and understanding. Embracing your true self means recognizing all parts of you—your strengths, weaknesses, desires, and fears.

These concepts can help you explore yourself more deeply and understand how you interact with others and the world. By reflecting on them, you can gain insights that support your personal growth and relationships.

The Creator

About Kim Aronson

I grew up in Copenhagen, Denmark, in the 1960s and '70s. As a child, I wasn't the best student. I could never sit still, and I think I would have probably been diagnosed with ADHD. I also didn't know at the time that I was dyslexic—no one did. I hated writing, and I couldn't make sense of any of the words I saw on the page. But if someone handed me some markers and glue, I was in heaven! I loved being creative, and this creativity provided me with a much-needed outlet for my other academic frustrations.

Throughout my life, I've always been an early adopter of technology. When I sat in front of a computer at an event in a Library in Copenhagen in 1995, where they were "showing off" the internet, I was *mesmerized*. After this, my first project using technology was creating customized icons that I sold at the local Mac store. A bit later, I started creating animations using Macromedia Director. Those moments became my first experiences of merging my creativity and technology. It allowed me to express myself without limits.

I created many online services in the late '90s and early 2000s, including a social network site in Denmark called Mandala. I also created a search site for spiritual seekers called ZenSearch, among many others.

However, the one that stuck around and became very successful was my online dating site, Soulmate, which I founded before creating a few other US-based dating sites over the next few years.

Although you've indeed just finished one of my books, I'm still not much of a writer. I love expressing myself and have always had many ideas and insights to share, but writing has been hard for me. This is why I've learned, over the last few years, all about the wonders of AI and LLM (Large Language Models). I have discovered how these programs can help me express my thoughts, feelings, and the wisdom I've accumulated over many years. It helps me communicate what's important to me and what I feel would be essential and helpful for others. As such, this book series has, to an extended degree, been created with the help of AI.

I hope you find the insights and exercises in this book and the rest of the series useful and inspiring. Please contact me with any thoughts, ideas, or wisdom to share. I would enjoy connecting.

www.WisdomManuals.com

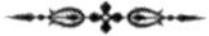

My professional website is: www.KimAronson.com
I offer intuitive readings to illuminate your path and provide clarity, personalized coaching sessions designed to empower you to reach your goals, and insightful teachings that will deepen your understanding of yourself and the world around you.